MY ANTI DEPRIME RITUALS
10 HAPPINESS BOOSTER ACTIONS

A study from McGill University, published in 2011 in Nature Neuroscience, shows how much music stimulates production dopamine, which causes a strong sense of well-being.
What if today we started the day by listening to our music favorite with pleasure in a cozy place and with a delicious tea or coffee ..

Month .... Year ....

Monday .... Week ....

TODAY WILL BE FANTASTIC!

MY 1 0 PURE HAPPINESS OF THE DAY ACTIVITIES

☐ .... ☐ ....

☐ .... ☐ ....

☐ .... ☐ ....

☐ .... ☐ ....

☐ .... ☐ ....

" The ' Darkness can not drive out ' dark, the only light can. Hate can not drive out hate, only the ' love the can. "
Martin Luther King

MY ANTI DEPRIME RITUALS
10 HAPPINESS BOOSTER ACTIONS

Daylight, via the hypothalamus, increases serotonin.
"It is all the more stimulating when we receive it early in the
morning",
points out Professor Lejoyeux, author of
"The four seasons of good humor" at
Pocket editions

Month .... Year ....

Tuesday .... Week ....

TODAY WILL BE FANTASTIC!

MY 10 PURE HAPPINESS OF THE DAY ACTIVITIES

☐ .... ☐ ....

☐ .... ☐ ....

☐ .... ☐ ....

☐ .... ☐ ....

☐ .... ☐ ....

" A well-defined goal is halfway achieved. "
Abraham Lincoln.

MY ANTI DEPRIME RITUALS
10 HAPPINESS BOOSTER ACTIONS

From the 1980s, Dr Henri Rubinstein, French neurologist,
explained that a minute of laughter was comparable to 45 minutes
of
relaxation. By laughing, the body releases the pressure of everyday
life and
releases endorphins, with antidepressant and anxiolytic effect.

Month .... Year ....

Wednesday.................Week ....

TODAY WILL BE FANTASTIC!

MY 1 0 PURE HAPPINESS OF THE DAY ACTIVITIES

☐ .... ☐ ....

☐ .... ☐ ....

☐ .... ☐ ....

☐ .... ☐ ....

☐ .... ☐ ....

*"Do not expect to be happy to smile. Smile instead
in order to be happy." - Edward L. Kramer "*

MY ANTI DEPRIME RITUALS
10 HAPPINESS BOOSTER ACTIONS

Other pillars of happiness according to neuroscience, adopt everything
that decreases your stress, such as meditation. "Practiced two times a week for two months, it lowers the rate of cortisol (stress hormone) in the blood and stimulates the production endorphin, serotonin and oxytocin, which is the hormone of emotional security and sociability, "explains the psychologist Jeanne Siaud-Facchin.

Month .... Year ....

Thursday .... Week ....

TODAY WILL BE FANTASTIC!

MY 1 0 PURE HAPPINESS OF THE DAY ACTIVITIES

- [ ] ....
- [ ] ....
- [ ] ....
- [ ] ....
- [ ] ....

- [ ] ....
- [ ] ....
- [ ] ....
- [ ] ....
- [ ] ....

" I have decided to be happy because c ' is good for health. "
" Voltaire "

MY ANTI DEPRIME RITUALS
10 HAPPINESS BOOSTER ACTIONS

And the hugs? "Twenty seconds is enough to get your dose oxytocin, the hormone of tenderness ", underlines Dr. Frédéric Saldmann, who suggests the hug before a meal for its effect appetite suppressant. We recommend this painless diet!
What happiness!

Month .... Year ....

Friday.................. Week ....

TODAY WILL BE FANTASTIC!

MY 1 0 PURE HAPPINESS OF THE DAY ACTIVITIES

☐ .... ☐ ....

☐ .... ☐ ....

☐ .... ☐ ....

☐ .... ☐ ....

☐ .... ☐ ....

" I now only want to collect the moments of happiness. ~ Stendhal "

MY ANTI DEPRIME RITUALS
10 HAPPINESS BOOSTER ACTIONS

Studies conducted by Stanford University show that
nature walks can not only make us more
happy, but also decrease our tendency to ruminate and
stir up negative thoughts!
Nature green power !!

Month .... Year ....

Saturday.................. Week ....

TODAY WILL BE FANTASTIC!

MY 1 0 PURE HAPPINESS OF THE DAY ACTIVITIES

☐ ....
☐ ....
☐ ....
☐ ....
☐ ....

☐ ....
☐ ....
☐ ....
☐ ....
☐ ....

" *Joy is like a river: nothing n ' stops its course.*

~

Henry Miller "

MY ANTI DEPRIME RITUALS
10 HAPPINESS BOOSTER ACTIONS

A few squares of chocolate is associated with an increase in dopamine according to a study published in 2013 in the journal Obesity.

Do not hesitate to nibble sparingly good chocolate, containing 70% cocoa, an important source of phenylethylamine (PEA), doping agent which causes the secretion of dopamine!

To eat chocolate !!!

Month .... Year ....

Sunday .... Week ....

TODAY WILL BE FANTASTIC!

MY 1 0 PURE HAPPINESS OF THE DAY ACTIVITIES

☐ .... ☐ ....

☐ .... ☐ ....

☐ .... ☐ ....

☐ .... ☐ ....

☐ .... ☐ ....

" Life is a mystery that ' we must live, not a problem solve. ~ Gandhi

MY ANTI DEPRIME RITUALS
10 HAPPINESS BOOSTER ACTIONS

A study from McGill University, published in 2011 in Nature Neuroscience, shows how much music stimulates production dopamine, which causes a strong sense of well-being.
What if today we started the day by listening to our music favorite with pleasure in a cozy place and with a delicious tea or coffee ..

Month .... Year ....

Monday .... Week ....

TODAY WILL BE FANTASTIC!

MY 1 0 PURE HAPPINESS OF THE DAY ACTIVITIES

☐ ....   ☐ ....

☐ ....   ☐ ....

☐ ....   ☐ ....

☐ ....   ☐ ....

☐ ....   ☐ ....

" The ' Darkness can not drive out ' dark, the only light can. Hate can not drive out hate, only the ' love the can. "
Martin Luther King

MY ANTI DEPRIME RITUALS
10 HAPPINESS BOOSTER ACTIONS

Daylight, via the hypothalamus, increases serotonin.
"It is all the more stimulating when we receive it early in the morning",
points out Professor Lejoyeux, author of
"The four seasons of good humor" at
Pocket editions

Month .... Year ....

Tuesday .... Week ....

TODAY WILL BE FANTASTIC!

MY 1 0 PURE HAPPINESS OF THE DAY ACTIVITIES

☐ .... ☐ ....

☐ .... ☐ ....

☐ .... ☐ ....

☐ .... ☐ ....

☐ .... ☐ ....

" A well-defined goal is halfway achieved. "
Abraham Lincoln.

MY ANTI DEPRIME RITUALS
10 HAPPINESS BOOSTER ACTIONS

From the 1980s, Dr Henri Rubinstein, French neurologist,
explained that a minute of laughter was comparable to 45 minutes
of
relaxation. By laughing, the body releases the pressure of everyday
life and
releases endorphins, with antidepressant and anxiolytic effect.

Month .... Year ....

Wednesday.................Week ....

TODAY WILL BE FANTASTIC!

MY 1 0 PURE HAPPINESS OF THE DAY ACTIVITIES

- [ ] ....
- [ ] ....
- [ ] ....
- [ ] ....
- [ ] ....

*"Do not expect to be happy to smile. Smile instead
in order to be happy."- Edward L. Kramer"*

MY ANTI DEPRIME RITUALS
10 HAPPINESS BOOSTER ACTIONS

Other pillars of happiness according to neuroscience, adopt everything
that decreases your stress, such as meditation. "Practiced two
times a week for two months, it lowers the rate of
cortisol (stress hormone) in the blood and stimulates the production
endorphin, serotonin and oxytocin, which is the hormone of
emotional security and sociability, "explains the psychologist
Jeanne Siaud-Facchin.

Month .... Year ....

Thursday .... Week ....

TODAY WILL BE FANTASTIC!

MY 1 0 PURE HAPPINESS OF THE DAY ACTIVITIES

☐ ....   ☐ ....

☐ ....   ☐ ....

☐ ....   ☐ ....

☐ ....   ☐ ....

☐ ....   ☐ ....

" I have decided to be happy because c ' is good for health. "
" Voltaire "

MY ANTI DEPRIME RITUALS
10 HAPPINESS BOOSTER ACTIONS

And the hugs? "Twenty seconds is enough to get your dose oxytocin, the hormone of tenderness ", underlines Dr. Frédéric Saldmann, who suggests the hug before a meal for its effect appetite suppressant. We recommend this painless diet! What happiness!

Month ....   Year ....

Friday..................   Week ....

TODAY WILL BE FANTASTIC!

MY 1 0 PURE HAPPINESS OF THE DAY ACTIVITIES

☐ ....   ☐ ....

☐ ....   ☐ ....

☐ ....   ☐ ....

☐ ....   ☐ ....

☐ ....   ☐ ....

" I now only want to collect the moments of happiness. ~ Stendhal "

MY ANTI DEPRIME RITUALS
10 HAPPINESS BOOSTER ACTIONS

Studies conducted by Stanford University show that
nature walks can not only make us more
happy, but also decrease our tendency to ruminate and
stir up negative thoughts!
Nature green power !!

Month .... Year ....

Saturday................... Week ....

TODAY WILL BE FANTASTIC!

MY 1 0 PURE HAPPINESS OF THE DAY ACTIVITIES

☐ .... ☐ ....

☐ .... ☐ ....

☐ .... ☐ ....

☐ .... ☐ ....

☐ .... ☐ ....

" *Joy is like a river: nothing n ' stops its course.*
~
Henry Miller "

MY ANTI DEPRIME RITUALS
10 HAPPINESS BOOSTER ACTIONS

A few squares of chocolate is associated with an increase in dopamine according to a study published in 2013 in the journal Obesity.

Do not hesitate to nibble sparingly good chocolate, containing 70% cocoa, an important source of phenylethylamine (PEA), doping agent which causes the secretion of dopamine!

To eat chocolate !!!

Month .... Year ....

Sunday .... Week ....

TODAY WILL BE FANTASTIC!

MY 1 0 PURE HAPPINESS OF THE DAY ACTIVITIES

☐ .... ☐ ....

☐ .... ☐ ....

☐ .... ☐ ....

☐ .... ☐ ....

☐ .... ☐ ....

" Life is a mystery that ' we must live, not a problem solve. ~ Gandhi

MY ANTI DEPRIME RITUALS
10 HAPPINESS BOOSTER ACTIONS

A study from McGill University, published in 2011 in Nature
Neuroscience, shows how much music stimulates production
dopamine, which causes a strong sense of well-being.
What if today we started the day by listening to our music
favorite with pleasure in a cozy place and with a delicious tea
or coffee ..

Month .... Year ....

Monday .... Week ....

TODAY WILL BE FANTASTIC!

MY 1 0 PURE HAPPINESS OF THE DAY ACTIVITIES

☐ ....   ☐ ....

☐ ....   ☐ ....

☐ ....   ☐ ....

☐ ....   ☐ ....

☐ ....   ☐ ....

" The ' Darkness can not drive out ' dark, the only light
can. Hate can not drive out hate, only the ' love the
can. "
Martin Luther King

MY ANTI DEPRIME RITUALS
10 HAPPINESS BOOSTER ACTIONS

Daylight, via the hypothalamus, increases serotonin.
"It is all the more stimulating when we receive it early in the
morning",
points out Professor Lejoyeux, author of
"The four seasons of good humor" at
Pocket editions

Month .... Year ....

Tuesday .... Week ....

TODAY WILL BE FANTASTIC!

MY 1 0 PURE HAPPINESS OF THE DAY ACTIVITIES

- ☐ ....
- ☐ ....
- ☐ ....
- ☐ ....
- ☐ ....

- ☐ ....
- ☐ ....
- ☐ ....
- ☐ ....
- ☐ ....

" A well-defined goal is halfway achieved. "
Abraham Lincoln.

MY ANTI DEPRIME RITUALS
10 HAPPINESS BOOSTER ACTIONS

From the 1980s, Dr Henri Rubinstein, French neurologist,
explained that a minute of laughter was comparable to 45 minutes
of
relaxation. By laughing, the body releases the pressure of everyday
life and
releases endorphins, with antidepressant and anxiolytic effect.

Month .... Year ....

Wednesday.................Week ....

TODAY WILL BE FANTASTIC!

MY 1 0 PURE HAPPINESS OF THE DAY ACTIVITIES

☐ .... ☐ ....

☐ .... ☐ ....

☐ .... ☐ ....

☐ .... ☐ ....

☐ .... ☐ ....

*"Do not expect to be happy to smile. Smile instead
in order to be happy." - Edward L. Kramer "*

MY ANTI DEPRIME RITUALS
10 HAPPINESS BOOSTER ACTIONS

Other pillars of happiness according to neuroscience, adopt everything
that decreases your stress, such as meditation. "Practiced two
times a week for two months, it lowers the rate of
cortisol (stress hormone) in the blood and stimulates the
production
endorphin, serotonin and oxytocin, which is the hormone of
emotional security and sociability, "explains the psychologist
Jeanne Siaud-Facchin.

Month .... Year ....

Thursday .... Week ....

TODAY WILL BE FANTASTIC!

MY 1 0 PURE HAPPINESS OF THE DAY ACTIVITIES

☐ .... ☐ ....

☐ .... ☐ ....

☐ .... ☐ ....

☐ .... ☐ ....

☐ .... ☐ ....

" I have decided to be happy because c ' is good for health. "
" Voltaire "

MY ANTI DEPRIME RITUALS
10 HAPPINESS BOOSTER ACTIONS

And the hugs? "Twenty seconds is enough to get your dose oxytocin, the hormone of tenderness ", underlines Dr. Frédéric Saldmann, who suggests the hug before a meal for its effect appetite suppressant. We recommend this painless diet! What happiness!

Month .... Year ....

Friday.................. Week ....

TODAY WILL BE FANTASTIC!

MY 1 0 PURE HAPPINESS OF THE DAY ACTIVITIES

☐ .... ☐ ....

☐ .... ☐ ....

☐ .... ☐ ....

☐ .... ☐ ....

☐ .... ☐ ....

"I now only want to collect the moments of happiness. ~ Stendhal"

MY ANTI DEPRIME RITUALS
10 HAPPINESS BOOSTER ACTIONS

Studies conducted by Stanford University show that
nature walks can not only make us more
happy, but also decrease our tendency to ruminate and
stir up negative thoughts!
Nature green power !!

Month .... Year ....

Saturday................... Week ....

TODAY WILL BE FANTASTIC!

MY 1 0 PURE HAPPINESS OF THE DAY ACTIVITIES

- [ ] ....
- [ ] ....
- [ ] ....
- [ ] ....
- [ ] ....

- [ ] ....
- [ ] ....
- [ ] ....
- [ ] ....
- [ ] ....

" *Joy is like a river: nothing n ' stops its course.*
~
Henry Miller "

MY ANTI DEPRIME RITUALS
10 HAPPINESS BOOSTER ACTIONS

A few squares of chocolate is associated with an increase in dopamine according to a study published in 2013 in the journal Obesity.

Do not hesitate to nibble sparingly good chocolate, containing 70% cocoa, an important source of phenylethylamine (PEA), doping agent which causes the secretion of dopamine!

To eat chocolate !!!

Month .... Year ....

Sunday .... Week ....

TODAY WILL BE FANTASTIC!

MY 1 0 PURE HAPPINESS OF THE DAY ACTIVITIES

- [ ] ....
- [ ] ....
- [ ] ....
- [ ] ....
- [ ] ....

- [ ] ....
- [ ] ....
- [ ] ....
- [ ] ....
- [ ] ....

" Life is a mystery that ' we must live, not a problem solve. ~ Gandhi

MY ANTI DEPRIME RITUALS
10 HAPPINESS BOOSTER ACTIONS

A study from McGill University, published in 2011 in Nature Neuroscience, shows how much music stimulates production dopamine, which causes a strong sense of well-being.
What if today we started the day by listening to our music favorite with pleasure in a cozy place and with a delicious tea or coffee ..

Month .... Year ....

Monday .... Week ....

TODAY WILL BE FANTASTIC!

MY 1 0 PURE HAPPINESS OF THE DAY ACTIVITIES

☐ .... ☐ ....

☐ .... ☐ ....

☐ .... ☐ ....

☐ .... ☐ ....

☐ .... ☐ ....

" The ' Darkness can not drive out ' dark, the only light can. Hate can not drive out hate, only the ' love the can. "
Martin Luther King

MY ANTI DEPRIME RITUALS
10 HAPPINESS BOOSTER ACTIONS

Daylight, via the hypothalamus, increases serotonin.
"It is all the more stimulating when we receive it early in the
morning",
points out Professor Lejoyeux, author of
"The four seasons of good humor" at
Pocket editions

Month .... Year ....

Tuesday .... Week ....

TODAY WILL BE FANTASTIC!

MY 1 0 PURE HAPPINESS OF THE DAY ACTIVITIES

☐ ....   ☐ ....

☐ ....   ☐ ....

☐ ....   ☐ ....

☐ ....   ☐ ....

☐ ....   ☐ ....

" A well-defined goal is halfway achieved. "
Abraham Lincoln.

MY ANTI DEPRIME RITUALS
10 HAPPINESS BOOSTER ACTIONS

From the 1980s, Dr Henri Rubinstein, French neurologist,
explained that a minute of laughter was comparable to 45 minutes
of
relaxation. By laughing, the body releases the pressure of everyday
life and
releases endorphins, with antidepressant and anxiolytic effect.

Month .... Year ....

Wednesday.................Week ....

TODAY WILL BE FANTASTIC!

MY 1 0 PURE HAPPINESS OF THE DAY ACTIVITIES

☐ .... ☐ ....

☐ .... ☐ ....

☐ .... ☐ ....

☐ .... ☐ ....

☐ .... ☐ ....

*" Do not expect to be happy to smile. Smile instead
in order to be happy. " - Edward L. Kramer "*

MY ANTI DEPRIME RITUALS
10 HAPPINESS BOOSTER ACTIONS

Other pillars of happiness according to neuroscience, adopt everything
that decreases your stress, such as meditation. "Practiced two
times a week for two months, it lowers the rate of
cortisol (stress hormone) in the blood and stimulates the production
endorphin, serotonin and oxytocin, which is the hormone of
emotional security and sociability, "explains the psychologist
Jeanne Siaud-Facchin.

Month .... Year ....

Thursday .... Week ....

TODAY WILL BE FANTASTIC!

MY 1 0 PURE HAPPINESS OF THE DAY ACTIVITIES

☐ ....   ☐ ....

☐ ....   ☐ ....

☐ ....   ☐ ....

☐ ....   ☐ ....

☐ ....   ☐ ....

" I have decided to be happy because c ' is good for health. "
" Voltaire "

MY ANTI DEPRIME RITUALS
10 HAPPINESS BOOSTER ACTIONS

And the hugs? "Twenty seconds is enough to get your dose oxytocin, the hormone of tenderness ", underlines Dr. Frédéric Saldmann, who suggests the hug before a meal for its effect appetite suppressant. We recommend this painless diet! What happiness!

Month .... Year ....

Friday................... Week ....

TODAY WILL BE FANTASTIC!

MY 1 0 PURE HAPPINESS OF THE DAY ACTIVITIES

☐ .... ☐ ....

☐ .... ☐ ....

☐ .... ☐ ....

☐ .... ☐ ....

☐ .... ☐ ....

" I now only want to collect the moments of happiness. ~ Stendhal "

MY ANTI DEPRIME RITUALS
10 HAPPINESS BOOSTER ACTIONS

Studies conducted by Stanford University show that
nature walks can not only make us more
happy, but also decrease our tendency to ruminate and
stir up negative thoughts!
Nature green power !!

Month .... Year ....

Saturday.................. Week ....

TODAY WILL BE FANTASTIC!

MY 1 0 PURE HAPPINESS OF THE DAY ACTIVITIES

- [ ] ....
- [ ] ....
- [ ] ....
- [ ] ....
- [ ] ....

- [ ] ....
- [ ] ....
- [ ] ....
- [ ] ....
- [ ] ....

" Joy is like a river: nothing n ' stops its course.
~
Henry Miller "

MY ANTI DEPRIME RITUALS
10 HAPPINESS BOOSTER ACTIONS

A few squares of chocolate is associated with an increase in dopamine according to a study published in 2013 in the journal Obesity.
Do not hesitate to nibble sparingly good chocolate, containing 70% cocoa, an important source of phenylethylamine (PEA), doping agent which causes the secretion of dopamine!
To eat chocolate !!!

Month .... Year ....

Sunday .... Week ....

TODAY WILL BE FANTASTIC!

MY 10 PURE HAPPINESS OF THE DAY ACTIVITIES

☐ .... ☐ ....

☐ .... ☐ ....

☐ .... ☐ ....

☐ .... ☐ ....

☐ .... ☐ ....

" Life is a mystery that ' we must live, not a problem solve. ~ Gandhi

MY ANTI DEPRIME RITUALS
10 HAPPINESS BOOSTER ACTIONS

A study from McGill University, published in 2011 in Nature
Neuroscience, shows how much music stimulates production
dopamine, which causes a strong sense of well-being.
What if today we started the day by listening to our music
favorite with pleasure in a cozy place and with a delicious tea
or coffee ..

Month .... Year ....

Monday .... Week ....

TODAY WILL BE FANTASTIC!

MY 1 0 PURE HAPPINESS OF THE DAY ACTIVITIES

- [ ] ....
- [ ] ....
- [ ] ....
- [ ] ....
- [ ] ....

" The ' Darkness can not drive out ' dark, the only light
can. Hate can not drive out hate, only the ' love the
can. "
Martin Luther King

MY ANTI DEPRIME RITUALS
10 HAPPINESS BOOSTER ACTIONS

Daylight, via the hypothalamus, increases serotonin.
"It is all the more stimulating when we receive it early in the morning",
points out Professor Lejoyeux, author of
"The four seasons of good humor" at
Pocket editions

Month .... Year ....

Tuesday .... Week ....

TODAY WILL BE FANTASTIC!

MY 1 0 PURE HAPPINESS OF THE DAY ACTIVITIES

☐ ....   ☐ ....

☐ ....   ☐ ....

☐ ....   ☐ ....

☐ ....   ☐ ....

☐ ....   ☐ ....

" A well-defined goal is halfway achieved. "
Abraham Lincoln.

MY ANTI DEPRIME RITUALS
10 HAPPINESS BOOSTER ACTIONS

From the 1980s, Dr Henri Rubinstein, French neurologist,
explained that a minute of laughter was comparable to 45 minutes
of
relaxation. By laughing, the body releases the pressure of everyday
life and
releases endorphins, with antidepressant and anxiolytic effect.

Month .... Year ....

Wednesday................Week ....

TODAY WILL BE FANTASTIC!

MY 1 0 PURE HAPPINESS OF THE DAY ACTIVITIES

- [ ] ....
- [ ] ....
- [ ] ....
- [ ] ....
- [ ] ....

- [ ] ....
- [ ] ....
- [ ] ....
- [ ] ....
- [ ] ....

*"Do not expect to be happy to smile. Smile instead
in order to be happy." - Edward L. Kramer "*

MY ANTI DEPRIME RITUALS
10 HAPPINESS BOOSTER ACTIONS

Other pillars of happiness according to neuroscience, adopt everything
that decreases your stress, such as meditation. "Practiced two
times a week for two months, it lowers the rate of
cortisol (stress hormone) in the blood and stimulates the production
endorphin, serotonin and oxytocin, which is the hormone of
emotional security and sociability, "explains the psychologist
Jeanne Siaud-Facchin.

Month .... Year ....

Thursday .... Week ....

TODAY WILL BE FANTASTIC!

MY 1 0 PURE HAPPINESS OF THE DAY ACTIVITIES

- [ ] ....
- [ ] ....
- [ ] ....
- [ ] ....
- [ ] ....

- [ ] ....
- [ ] ....
- [ ] ....
- [ ] ....
- [ ] ....

" I have decided to be happy because c ' is good for health. "
" Voltaire "

MY ANTI DEPRIME RITUALS
10 HAPPINESS BOOSTER ACTIONS

And the hugs? "Twenty seconds is enough to get your dose oxytocin, the hormone of tenderness ", underlines Dr. Frédéric Saldmann, who suggests the hug before a meal for its effect appetite suppressant. We recommend this painless diet!
What happiness!

Month .... Year ....

Friday.................. Week ....

TODAY WILL BE FANTASTIC!

MY 1 0 PURE HAPPINESS OF THE DAY ACTIVITIES

☐ .... ☐ ....

☐ .... ☐ ....

☐ .... ☐ ....

☐ .... ☐ ....

☐ .... ☐ ....

" I now only want to collect the moments of happiness. ~ Stendhal "

MY ANTI DEPRIME RITUALS
10 HAPPINESS BOOSTER ACTIONS

Studies conducted by Stanford University show that
nature walks can not only make us more
happy, but also decrease our tendency to ruminate and
stir up negative thoughts!
Nature green power !!

Month .... Year ....

Saturday.................. Week ....

TODAY WILL BE FANTASTIC!

MY 1 0 PURE HAPPINESS OF THE DAY ACTIVITIES

- [ ] ....
- [ ] ....
- [ ] ....
- [ ] ....
- [ ] ....

- [ ] ....
- [ ] ....
- [ ] ....
- [ ] ....
- [ ] ....

" *Joy is like a river: nothing n ' stops its course.*
~
Henry Miller "

MY ANTI DEPRIME RITUALS
10 HAPPINESS BOOSTER ACTIONS

A few squares of chocolate is associated with an increase in dopamine according to a study published in 2013 in the journal Obesity.

Do not hesitate to nibble sparingly good chocolate, containing 70% cocoa, an important source of phenylethylamine (PEA), doping agent which causes the secretion of dopamine!

To eat chocolate !!!

Month .... Year ....

Sunday .... Week ....

TODAY WILL BE FANTASTIC!

MY 1 0 PURE HAPPINESS OF THE DAY ACTIVITIES

☐ .... ☐ ....

☐ .... ☐ ....

☐ .... ☐ ....

☐ .... ☐ ....

☐ .... ☐ ....

" Life is a mystery that ' we must live, not a problem solve. ~ Gandhi